Dash Diet for Blood Pressure

Quick and Easy Recipes and Meal Plans to Naturally Lower Blood Pressure and Reduce Hypertension

Dana Dittman

Table of Contents

Introduction

Is your physical health not in the best of shape? When I say this, I don't just refer to your muscle mass or the type of body build you currently have. I'm referring more to the various internal factors within your body, specifically your blood pressure. This is defined as how much blood is pushing against the walls of blood vessels. It's the job of your heart to pump your blood inside your blood vessels to transport it across your body. However, there's always the risk of developing high blood pressure, also known as hypertension, which can make it harder for your heart to properly pump blood throughout your body. If you happen to struggle with high blood pressure, you may end up with harmful health conditions like atherosclerosis, kidney disease, hardened arteries, and strokes—or your heart may end up failing. According to a WebMD article titled *Causes of High Blood Pressure* (Beckerman, 2021), a normal amount of blood pressure to sustain is 120 over 80. Here are some other blood pressure ranges to consider: 120–129 over 80 is elevated blood pressure; 130–139 over 80–89 is Stage 1 high blood pressure; 140 and higher over 90 and higher is Stage 2 high blood pressure; and anything higher than 180 over anything higher than 120 is a hypertension crisis, which requires a trip to a doctor.

One article for *Healthline* clarifies that the first number of these combinations represents your *systolic* blood pressure, while the second represents your *diastolic* blood pressure. Your systolic blood pressure measures the force of your blood flowing against artery walls while the ventricles of your heart push blood throughout your whole body. Meanwhile, your diastolic blood pressure measures the force of your blood while your heart relaxes and its ventricles refill with blood. It's very important to have both high and low blood pressure monitored and managed, though the former is much more common. Nearly half of all adults in the United States have high blood pressure, as stated by the American College of Cardiology (McDermott, 2019).

One risk factor that contributes to high blood pressure is gender. It was diagnosed by the American Heart Association that men have a higher risk of increased blood pressure than women until they become 64 years old. However, women are at higher risk than men as soon as they reach 65 years of age. You also place yourself in danger of developing higher blood pressure by not getting in enough physical activity or if your daily diet is high in fats and sugars.

There are many other factors that contribute to increased blood pressure, with some of the most notable being stress, high cholesterol, smoking, having relatives with known high blood pressure issues, and an overabundance of salt in your diet. Those with heightened blood pressure are very sensitive to salt, which means if they consume more than the minimum amount of salt they need, it only further raises their blood pressure (Beckerman, 2021). In this book, there are several different kinds of recipes both easy and quick to prepare for yourself and can help prevent your blood pressure from going through the roof. By following along with the meal plans and recipes discussed in this book, you'll be able to make nutritious dishes that will help gradually lower your blood pressure and reduce the risk of hypertension. I have a passion for fast diets to manage blood pressure, which drove me to compile this book to help others improve their own health.

One of the most effective ways to decrease your blood pressure is to consume less salt. Another useful tip is to include more fruits and vegetables high in potassium in your daily diet, such as raisins, bananas, mangoes, tomatoes, bok choy, and kale. Eating whole grains like oats and brown rice is another great way to lower your blood pressure. Some research done by the Physicians Committee for Responsible Medicine (PCRM) explains how a mainly plant-based diet can lower your levels of blood pressure—and therefore, your risk of conditions like heart failure. Benefits like this are why it can be a great decision to make healthy changes to your everyday diet. PCRM also brings up how an analytic study done by authors Yoko Yokoyama and Kunihiro Nishimura revealed a strong link between vegetarian diets and normal levels of blood pressure. During this study, individuals with a vegetarian diet had lower blood pressure levels than those who had more meat in their diets (Yokoyama, Nishimura, 2014). Overall, this study stresses the importance of changing up one's diet to improve their own blood pressure and decrease the risk of hypertension or other health-related concerns.

Some other useful tips in treating your high blood pressure include omitting any unhealthy foods from your regular diet, drinking more water, partaking in more physical activities like exercise, keeping a consistent and healthy weight, finding good ways to manage your stress levels, and monitoring your blood pressure throughout your day. It's also a good idea to stop taking medicines such as diet pills or medications for ADHD and colds as these can contribute to raising your blood pressure. If that's the case, you'll have to either stop taking the medication, change your daily dosage, or swap it out for a new one. However, there may be situations where you may need to be prescribed certain blood pressure medications if you suffer from conditions like Stage 2 hypertension. Some of these prescriptions include calcium channel blockers, diuretics, and angiotensin-converting enzyme inhibitors (McDermott, 2019).

PCRM also mentions a review of the journal *Progress in Cardiovascular Diseases* that discusses how people with vegetarian eating habits have better heart health. Further research showed lengthy evidence for plant-based diets and their ability to cut back blood pressure, along with a few other additional benefits. These include a 40% reduction of heart disease risk, partially or fully opened arteries, a 34% reduction of hypertension risk, a decrease in cholesterol levels, and loss in weight. Plant-based dietary routines are helpful, as the types of foods included in them contain plenty of phytonutrients like lycopene or carotenoids. These kinds of phytonutrients are vital for reducing any inflammation in your body. Many meat products, however, tend to be packed with cholesterol, saturated fat, and even environmental pollutants that are hazardous to your heart health. PCRM Clinical Research Director Hana Kahleova states how a diet based mainly in plants or vegetable products can reverse heart disease as well as prevent it. Some notes taken from this research elaborate on how adopting a healthier diet lowers the chances of having a heart attack by 81% to 94%. This is different from most medications, which only cut the probability down by 20% to 30%.

Overall, taking up a diet based mostly on fruits and vegetables is healthy for you, because the high potassium amounts they have can lower blood pressure. Plant-based diets can also be great for your overall health, due to how little sodium they contain. If you want to reduce your high blood pressure, or maintain the healthy levels you already have, then it's important to cut back or avoid any dishes or products with meat or dairy included. Doing so can decrease the thickness of your blood, making it easier for your heart to pump and decrease blood pressure. PCRM also mentions another analysis done by Dr. Thomas Semlitsch, which states that reducing the amount of sodium in your diet can also lower systolic blood pressure by 3.6 mmHg. To do this, it's important to avoid or limit how much processed food you eat. This also counts towards snacks, dairy, and canned foods. Decrease how much sodium-filled products you use in whatever meals you cook and switch them out in favor of veggies, fruits, and grains. If you want a good idea of what kinds of dishes you can make to decrease your own blood pressure, then read on to the next chapter to look over some of the healthiest dinners you can cook in a short amount of time.

Chapter 1:

Healthy Dinner Ideas

If you're currently suffering from high blood pressure, then you likely feel its effects and negative impact on your health throughout your day. Fortunately, there are plenty of recipes you can try out to help naturally lower your blood pressure. This chapter will go over plenty of healthy dinner recipes that are both easy and quick to put together, which means less work and stress for you to worry about. There is a nearly endless variety of options out there for you to choose from, many of which have different benefits and features that cater towards individuals with specific dietary requirements. But many of these dishes help to improve other parts of your body, as well as being high in protein or fiber.

Chickpea and Quinoa Grain Bowl

Our first recipe is the *chickpea and quinoa grain bowl*, which is high in fiber and dairy-free. The following ingredients are needed to make this nutritious meal:

- 1 cup of cooked quinoa
- ⅓ cup of canned chickpeas

- ½ cup of sliced cucumbers

- ½ cup of sliced cherry tomatoes

- ¼ diced avocados

- 3 tablespoons of hummus

- 1 teaspoon of chopped parsley

- 1 tablespoon of chopped roasted red peppers

- 1 tablespoon of water

- 1 tablespoon of lemon juice

- 1 pinch of ground pepper and salt

Once you've gathered all the necessary ingredients, place the quinoa, cucumbers, avocado, tomatoes, and chickpeas into a large bowl. Afterwards, place the water, lemon juice, hummus, and red peppers into another bowl and stir them together to make dressing. You'll probably need to add a little more water to the dressing to reach the right level of consistency. Throw in some salt, ground pepper, and parsley into the mix and serve the dressing next to the bowl. The final step is to enjoy the healthy meal you've whipped up.

Skillet Steak and Mushroom Sauce

Another recipe to help diminish high blood pressure is the *skillet steak and mushroom sauce*, which takes under 25 minutes to cook. Here's a list of all the ingredients you'll require:

- ¾ pound of boneless beef top sirloin steak
- 2 teaspoons of salt-free steak grilling seasoning
- ¾ cups of trimmed broccoli rabe
- 2 teaspoons of canola oil
- 3 cups of sliced mushrooms
- 2 cups of frozen peas
- ¼ teaspoon of salt
- 2 teaspoons of cornstarch
- 1 cup of unsalted beef broth
- 1 tablespoon of whole-grain mustard

After getting your ingredients, preheat your oven to 350 degrees Fahrenheit and sprinkle the steak seasoning onto the meat. Then, heat up your canola oil to medium-high in a 12-inch cast-iron skillet, and throw in your meat and broccoli rabe while it's heating up. Cook your concoction for 4 minutes; turn your broccoli rabe just once, but leave the meat alone. As the meat is cooking, place the frozen peas around it.

Next, move the skillet over to your oven and bake the meal for exactly 8 minutes or until the meat is cooked to medium-rare. Take your meat and veggies out of the skillet before covering it up and keeping it warm. Don't discard your skillet yet: Your next task is to make the sauce for the steak. First, add the sliced mushrooms to the leftover drippings inside the skillet. Heat them up over medium-high heat for about 3 minutes, while stirring them around.

Use a whisk to mix the mustard, salt, beef broth, and cornstarch into the mushrooms. Let the sauce cook until you see it bubble up and thicken in texture. Keep stirring and cooking for another minute. Then you can serve your hearty sauce with your warm steak and vegetables.

Veggie and Hummus Sandwich

Another scrumptious recipe that can decrease your blood pressure is a simple *veggie and hummus sandwich*. You can interchange some of your own favorite vegetables or types of hummus to make the sandwich of your choosing. All the basic ingredients you'll need to put together this sandwich is:

- 2 slices of whole-grain bread
- ¼ of a mashed avocado
- ¼ cup of sliced cucumbers
- ¼ sliced medium-sized red bell peppers
- ¼ cup of shredded carrots
- ¼ cup of mixed salad greens

The next step is fairly quick and simple: Spread one bread slice with hummus and one with mashed avocado, and then stack up all the veggies together. You can either eat the sandwich whole or slice it up in halves: The choice is yours! This option is not only low in calories and sodium, but is also great for boosting your immunity system.

Cheeseburger-Stuffed Baked Potatoes

Are you craving a burger at the moment but don't want to make your high blood pressure worse? Then the recipe for *cheeseburger-stuffed baked potatoes* might be a healthier substitute to both appease your appetite and improve your health. This recipe is free of any gluten that would come from ingredients like hamburger buns and is healthy for your heart. Here are the key ingredients you'll need to cobble this dinner together:

- ½ pound of cooked ground beef

- 4 teaspoons of cheese (chef's choice)

- ½ cup of shredded iceberg lettuce

- ½ cup of diced tomatoes

- ½ cup of sliced red onions

- 4 medium-sized russet potatoes

- ½ cup of low-fat mayo

The three-step process to put this healthy meal together is straightforward and easy to follow. First, pierce the potatoes with a fork before microwaving them on a medium setting for about 20 minutes. Make sure to turn them around every so often. If you don't prefer a microwave, you can place the potatoes inside your oven and bake them for 45 minutes to 1 hour at 425 degrees Fahrenheit. After your potatoes are all cooked, move them over to a cutting board to let them cool off.

Second, cut lengthwise across each of the potatoes, but don't cut entirely through them, and pinch both of their ends to expose the skin. It's a good idea to use a towel or mitts to keep your hands from being burned. Finally, once it's cut open, top the warm potatoes with the beef, greens, and other ingredients and dig in while they're hot.

One-Pot Garlicky Shrimp and Spinach

There is also a recipe for a dish of *one-pot garlicky shrimp and spinach*. This recipe takes little time to make and is free of any eggs, nuts, and soy for those who have specific allergies. Use the following ingredients to put this healthy dish together:

- 1 pound of deveined and peeled shrimp

- 10 cups of spinach

- 1 tablespoon of chopped parsley

- 6 medium-sized cloves of sliced garlic

- 1 tablespoon of lemon juice

- 1 ½ teaspoons of lemon zest

- **¼ teaspoon of salt with an additional ⅛ teaspoon set aside**

- ¼ teaspoon of crushed red peppers

- 3 separate tablespoons of extra-virgin olive oil

Heat up only 1 tablespoon of olive oil in a large pot above a medium heat setting. Then throw in half of the garlic cloves and keep cooking for about 1 to 2 minutes, until the garlic begins to turn brown.

Next, include the spinach and ¼ teaspoon of salt and toss the mixture around to properly coat it. Continue cooking the mixture for 3 to 5 minutes while occasionally stirring it until the spinach inside starts to wilt. Afterwards, remove the pot from heat and add in the lemon juice. Stir it around before moving the mixture into a large bowl and warming the pot back up.

Next, increase the heat to medium-high and put the last 2 tablespoons of olive oil into the pot. Once that's done, be sure to include the rest of the garlic and cook the mixture for another 1 to 2 minutes until it browns. As soon as it reaches that point, throw in the shrimp, crushed red peppers, and the ⅛ teaspoon of salt you set aside earlier.

Stir everything together thoroughly for about 3 to 5 more minutes until the shrimp is cooked all the way. Finally, place the shrimp on top of the cooked spinach and sprinkle it all with the parsley and lemon zest.

Spicy Chicken and Snow Pea Skillet

One other good recipe you can try to lower your blood pressure is the *spicy chicken and snow pea skillet*. This dinner option is low in calories and sodium, along with being rich in protein. Here are the ingredients you'll need to put this dish together:

- 1 to 2 teaspoons of harissa paste
- 1 ½ cups of trimmed snow pea pods
- 2 cups of halved cherry tomatoes
- 2 cloves of minced garlic
- 1 tablespoon of extra-virgin olive oil
- ½ cup of reduced sodium chicken broth
- 15 ounces of no-salt added chickpeas (garbanzo beans)
- ¼ teaspoon of salt
- ⅓ cup of parsley
- 1 lemon
- ¼ cup plain fat-free Greek yogurt

- four 1-ounce slices of French bread (optional)
- ¼ cup of pitted and halved Kalamata olives
- 1 pound of skinless and boneless chicken breast halves, cut into ¾ inch pieces

To start off, place the chicken, garlic, and harissa paste into a medium-sized bowl and toss it around to coat. Then heat up the olive oil in a 12-inch skillet, with a medium-high setting.

Next, add the chicken and cook and stir it around until it's no longer pink in color, and take it out of the skillet. Once you've done that, mix together the snow peas, chicken broth, garbanzo beans, and salt inside the skillet. Raise the temperature until it starts to boil and then lower the heat. Cover up the mixture and let it simmer for 5 minutes or until the pea pods tenderize and the tomatoes begin to soften up.

At this stage, bring the chicken back to the skillet. The last step is to remove 1 teaspoon of zest and squeeze 1 tablespoon of juice directly from the lemon. Stir the lemon juice and zest together, along with the olives and parsley into the chicken concoction. Serve the finished dish with Greek yogurt and bread for dipping if you want.

Mixed Greens With Lentils and Apple Slices

If you're looking for a healthy meal that includes a taste of fruit, then a classic dish of *mixed greens with lentils and apple slices* may be the perfect choice for you. This meal is ideal for vegetarians and has the additional benefits of support for aging and your immune system. Here is a list of all the ingredients you'll need to put together this quick dish:

- 1 ½ cups mixed salad greens
- 1 apple to slice up
- ½ a cup of cooked lentils
- 1 tablespoon of red wine vinegar
- 1 ½ tablespoons of crumbled feta cheese
- 2 teaspoons of extra-virgin olive oil

The process for preparing this meal is relatively simple: all you need to do is to mix the lentils and greens together, throw in the feta crumbles and half of the apple slices, and drizzle the mixture with olive oil and vinegar. The rest of the apple slices can be enjoyed as a side dish.

Stuffed Sweet Potato With Hummus Dressing

A *stuffed sweet potato with hummus dressing* is another nutritious dinner choice to decrease blood pressure. This meal can provide support for both your heart health and your wellbeing during pregnancy. It also requires only five ingredients to cook, making it easier and less time-consuming for your overall schedule:

- 1 large scrubbed sweet potato
- ¼ cup of hummus
- 1 cup of rinsed black beans
- 2 tablespoons of water
- ¾ cup of chopped kale

Your first step is to poke your sweet potato with a fork and microwave it for 7 to 10 minutes until it's completely cooked. While that's busy cooking, wash and drain your kale to let the water attach to the leaves.

Put the rinsed kale in a medium-sized saucepan, cover the pan, and let it cook on a medium-high setting. Stir the kale around occasionally until it begins to wilt up. Throw in the black beans once it does, and a few tablespoons of water as well if the pan is dry. Keep cooking and stirring this mixture for 1 to 2 minutes or until it starts to steam.

Your last step is to split the sweet potato open and place the bean and kale mixture on top of it. Afterwards, mix the ¼ cup of hummus and 2 tablespoons of water together in a small side dish: Use as much water as needed for the dressing to become consistent enough. Finally, drizzle this dressing on top of the stuffed potato and dig in!

Charred Shrimp, Pesto, and Quinoa

Do you happen to be a fan of seafood, but are looking for a dish that relieves blood pressure? Look no further than this delicious recipe for a bowl of *charred shrimp, pesto, and quinoa.* This dish takes less than half an hour to put together. It can improve bone health and you can add or swap out some of the ingredients to suit your dietary needs. Here's a list of everything you'll need to prepare this hearty dinner:

- 1 pound of large peeled and deveined shrimp

- ⅓ cup of pesto

- 2 cups of cooked quinoa

- 1 tablespoon of extra-virgin olive oil

- 2 tablespoons of balsamic vinegar

- ¼ teaspoon of ground pepper

- ½ a teaspoon of salt

- 4 cups of arugula

- 1 diced avocado

- 1 cup of halved cherry tomatoes

The process to make this healthy dish consists of only three main steps. First, use a whisk to mix together the olive oil, salt, pepper, vinegar, and pesto in a big bowl. Once this is done, take out 4 tablespoons of this new vinaigrette into a smaller bowl and move both bowls aside for now.

Your next step is to warm up a large cast-iron skillet on a medium-high setting. Heat up the shrimp for 4 to 5 minutes, stirring every now and then, until they cook with a slight char. As soon as the shrimp is cooked all the way, place them onto a separate plate.

Lastly, throw the quinoa and arugula into the large vinaigrette bowl, tossing them around for a proper coating. Then split this up into four smaller bowls, topping each one with the shrimp, tomatoes, and diced avocados. All that's left is to drizzle the four bowls with 1 tablespoon each of the pesto sauce.

Pan-Seared Steak With Crispy Herbs and Escarole

Here's another recipe that's great for lovers of both vegetables and meat: *pan-seared steak with crispy herbs and escarole.* This dish may suit you if you're looking for an option that only takes about 20 minutes to make and doesn't require much cleanup. It has added perks of being free of any sugars, gluten, or carbohydrates. Everything you'll need to prepare this dish for your dinners includes the following:

- 1 pound of sirloin steak (roughly ½ an inch thick)
- 16 cups of chopped escarole
- 1 sprig of rosemary
- 5 sprigs of thyme
- 3 sprigs of sage
- 4 crushed garlic cloves
- ½ teaspoon of salt, split in half
- ½ teaspoon of ground pepper, split in half
- 2 tablespoons of canola or grapeseed oil

(A sprig is a 2 to 4-inch piece of whatever herb you need for your dish.)

First up, sprinkle the first half of the ½ teaspoon of salt and pepper onto your steak, before cooking it in a big cast-iron skillet on a medium-high setting for roughly 3 minutes.

Second, turn the steak over to add the crushed garlic, sage, rosemary, thyme, and oil. Once that's finished, stir the herbs around every few moments for 3 to 4 minutes until an instant-read thermometer placed in the thickest area of the meat reaches 125 degrees Fahrenheit, meaning the steak is now medium-rare.

After the steak finishes cooking, move it onto a plate and put the herbs and garlic on top of it, before placing foil over it. Then place the chopped escarole and the other half of the ½ teaspoon of salt and pepper onto the skillet and cook and stir for about 2 minutes or until the escarole wilts. Cut the steak into thin slices, serve it with the cooked escarole and herbs on the side, and savor your hard work.

Tomato, Cucumber, and White Bean Salad With Basil Vinaigrette

If you're craving a dish abundant with vegetables, you might like the recipe for a *tomato, cucumber, and white bean salad with basil vinaigrette*. This dish also requires little effort to clean up, so that's another added bonus. Take a look at the different ingredients you'll need to put this salad together:

- ½ cup of packed basil leaves
- 10 cups of mixed greens
- 1 cup of sliced cucumbers
- ¼ cup of extra-virgin olive oil
- 1 tablespoon of chopped shallot

- 3 tablespoons of red wine vinegar

- ¼ teaspoon of salt

- ¼ teaspoon of ground pepper

- 1 teaspoon of honey

- 2 teaspoons of Dijon mustard

- 15 ounces of rinsed low-sodium cannellini beans

- 1 cup of halved grape or cherry tomatoes

This recipe only requires a few small steps to make. You first need to put the basil leaves, shallot, honey, mustard, olive oil, vinegar, salt, and pepper inside of a miniature food processor. Turn the device on and let the food mixture process until it becomes smooth. Dump the mixture into a large bowl before adding in the mixed greens, sliced cucumbers, tomatoes, and cannellini beans on top of it. Toss the salad around to fully coat the ingredients and enjoy your creation!

Grilled Salmon With Vegetables

If you're looking for a nutritious dish with fish, then a simple *grilled salmon with vegetables* is a great option to lower your blood pressure. Have a gander at all the ingredients you'll need to put this meal together to boost your health:

- 1 ¼ pound of salmon filet (sliced into 4 equal portions)

- 2 red or orange or yellow bell peppers (halved, trimmed, and seeded)

- ½ teaspoon of salt, separated into ¼ teaspoons

- ½ teaspoon of ground pepper

- 1 medium zucchini cut lengthwise

- 1 medium-sized red onion sliced into 1-inch wedges

- 1 lemon cut into 4 wedges

- 1 tablespoon of olive oil

- ¼ cup of thinly sliced basil

Before you get started, make sure to preheat your grill to a medium-high setting. Then brush your zucchini, onion wedges, and peppers with olive oil and sprinkle ¼ teaspoon of salt over them. Afterwards, sprinkle the salmon filet with pepper and the other ¼ teaspoon of salt.

Your next task is to put all the veggies and salmon portions with their skin-sides facing down onto the grill. Heat up the vegetables while turning them around a few times, spending 4 to 6 minutes on each side, until grill marks start to show up.

Next, cook the salmon filets for 8 to 10 minutes without turning them until they start to flake, and test them with a fork. Once they've cooled down enough, chop up the vegetables and throw them all into a large bowl. The next step is to deskin the salmon filets, but you're free to eat them with the skin if you so choose.

Regardless, take the salmon from the grill and serve them along with the grilled vegetables. Finally, garnish each of the servings with a lemon wedge and 1 tablespoon of basil each. You can also round out this hearty dish with a side of quinoa or brown rice.

Seared Scallops With White Bean Ragu and Charred Lemon

Another tasty and healthy dinner with seafood includes a helping of *seared scallops with white bean ragu and charred lemon*. You'll need the following ingredients to assemble this particular dish:

- 1 pound of dry sea scallops (with their muscle sides removed)
- 10 cups of thinly sliced white chard or mature spinach
- 1 lemon cut in half
- 2 minced garlic cloves
- 3 divided teaspoons of olive oil
- ½ divided teaspoon of ground pepper

- 1 cup of low-sodium chicken broth

- 1 tablespoon of rinsed and chopped capers

- 1 tablespoon of butter

- 15 ounces of rinsed and drained low-sodium cannellini beans

- 2 tablespoons of chopped parsley

- ⅓ cup of dry white wine

While buying the needed ingredients, it's important to specifically look for dry scallops because some are drenched in a solution that doesn't let them sear properly while cooking.

First, heat up 2 of the teaspoons of olive oil in a big skillet over medium-high heat. Then toss in the greens, cook, and stir for roughly 4 minutes until they wilt up.

Afterwards, throw in the capers, minced garlic, and ¼ teaspoon of pepper. Cook the mixture and stir it around for 30 seconds or until it becomes fragrant. Then throw in the beans, white wine, and chicken broth before bringing the entire concoction to a simmer. Lower the heat to keep a steady simmer and cover the skillet; keep cooking it for the next 5 minutes.

Then, you must remove the skillet from the heat and stir in 1 tablespoon of butter, and then cover it back up to keep it warm. As the mixture continues to cook, sprinkle the last ¼ teaspoon of ground pepper onto the dry scallops.

Heat up the last teaspoon of olive oil in a large nonstick skillet over another medium-high flame. Throw in the scallops after that and cook them for exactly 4 minutes or until both of their sides are browned. Once they're brown, put the cooked scallops onto a new plate.

Next, add the two lemon halves to the skillet with the cut-sides facing down, heat them up for 2 minutes until they're charred, and cut into the wedges. Finally, sprinkle the chopped parsley onto the sea scallops and bean ragu and serve them along with the charred lemon wedges.

Beef and Bean Sloppy Joes

Do you like sloppy joes? If yes, then you might like a tasty substitute of *beef and bean sloppy joes*. This recipe not only helps decrease blood pressure, but it also provides a high amount of fiber and health for your heart. To cook up this amazing dish, here's everything you'll require:

- ¾ pound of 90% lean ground beef
- 4 whole-wheat hamburger buns (toasted, if desired)
- 1 cup of sodium-free black beans
- 2 teaspoons of New Mexico chile powder
- 1 cup of sodium-free tomato sauce

- 1 tablespoon of olive oil
- 1 cup of chopped onions
- ½ teaspoon of garlic powder
- ½ teaspoon of onion powder
- 1 tablespoon of reduced-sodium Worcestershire sauce
- 1 pinch of cayenne pepper
- 3 tablespoons of ketchup
- 2 teaspoons of spicy brown mustard
- 1 teaspoon of light brown sugar

To make these sloppy joes, you first need to heat up the olive oil in a big nonstick skillet over medium-high heat. Then toss in the ground beef and cook it for 3 to 4 minutes, while breaking it apart with a wooden spoon until it turns a light shade of brown, but don't completely cook through it yet.

Next, use a slotted spoon to move the beef over to a new medium-sized bowl, so that the drippings can be preserved inside the skillet for later use. Once you've done that, throw the black beans and onions into the skillet; cook and stir the mixture around for 5 minutes or until the onions begin to soften.

The next step is to add all the powders into the skillet: garlic, onion, chile, and cayenne together. Heat up and stir the mixture for 30 seconds. After that, stir in the brown sugar, ketchup, mustard, tomato sauce, and

Worcestershire sauce. Bring the warm beef from the medium bowl back into the skillet before bringing the heat to a simmer.

Cook and stir the combined mixture for the next 5 minutes, until the ground beef is thoroughly cooked and the sauce is thickened. Finally, serve the beef on the whole-wheat buns and you're good to go.

Chinese Ginger Beef Stir-Fry With Baby Bok Choy

If you're looking for a meal to help decrease blood pressure, but you're also a fan of Chinese food, then you might enjoy making *Chinese ginger beef stir-fry with baby bok choy*. To get started, here's a list of all the essential ingredients you'll need to put this dinner together:

- ¾ pounds of trimmed beef steak
- 8 cups of baby bok choy (trimmed and cut into 2-inch pieces)
- 1 tablespoon of minced ginger
- 1 teaspoon and 1 divided tablespoon of dry sherry
- 1 ½ teaspoons of reduced-sodium soy sauce
- 1 tablespoon of vegetable oil

- 1 teaspoon of toasted sesame oil
- 1 teaspoon of cornstarch
- 3 tablespoons of unsalted chicken broth
- 2 tablespoons of oyster-flavored sauce

As you search for your ingredients, a great choice for your oyster sauce is the Lee Kum Kee Premium brand, as it contains the most concentrated flavor of oyster for your dish.

The first step to making the dish is to cut up the beef steak across the grain into 2-inch wide strips before cutting each of them across the grain into smaller, ¼ thick slices.

Then, mix the beef, soy sauce, ginger, cornstarch, and the 1 teaspoon of sherry into a medium-sized bowl. Keep stirring the mixture until you can't see the cornstarch anymore. Once that's finished, throw in the sesame oil until the beef becomes lightly coated with it.

The next step is to mix the oyster-flavored sauce and the last tablespoon of sherry into a smaller bowl and leave it alone for the moment. Afterwards, heat up either a 12-inch stainless steel skillet or 14-inch flat-bottomed, carbon-steel wok over a high flame until water evaporates on it after 1 to 2 seconds.

Swirl in the vegetable oil before adding the beef in an even layer. Let the meat cook for 1 minute and don't touch it until it takes on a brown color. As soon as it does, use a metal spatula to stir-fry it for 30 seconds to

1 minute until it turns light brown, but don't cook it all the way through.

Move the beef to a new plate and place the bok choy and chicken broth into the wok or skillet (whichever you decide to use). Cover it up and let it cook for 1 to 2 minutes until the bok choy becomes bright green and all of the residual liquid has been completely absorbed.

Put the beef back into the skillet or wok, throw in the leftover sauce, and stir-fry the mixture for 30 seconds to a minute, or at least until the bok choy is tender and the beef finishes cooking through.

Lamb and Eggplant Ragu

If you're in the mood for a healthy dinner that's Mediterranean-style, then a good choice for you is the *lamb and eggplant ragu*. This meal helps to improve your aging, immune system, and heart health. The following is an extensive list of the ingredients you'll need to cook this meal:

- 1 cup of whole-wheat penne/rigatoni/rotini

- 1 ½ cups of diced eggplant

- ¼ pounds of lean ground beef or ground lamb

- 2 cloves of chopped garlic

- 1 teaspoon of olive oil

- ¼ teaspoon of fennel seed

- 8 ounces of sodium-free tomato sauce

- ¼ teaspoon of salt

- ¼ teaspoon of ground pepper

- ½ a cup of red wine

- 1 teaspoon of toasted pine nuts

- 1 ½ teaspoons of chopped fresh oregano or ½ teaspoon of dried oregano

- ¼ cup of crumbled feta (optional)

Before you start cooking, boil a large pot of water. Boil the pasta for 8 to 10 minutes, based on what the package directions state.

While the pasta is boiling, cook the lamb or beef, fennel seed, and chopped garlic inside a large nonstick skillet over medium-high heat for 3 to 4 minutes. Break the meat apart with the back of a spoon in the meantime until it becomes more brown in color.

Then add in the olive oil and eggplants to cook for 4 minutes and occasionally stir it until the latter also becomes brown. After that, toss in the red wine and tomato sauce to cook and stir for 3 minutes.

Once the sauce thickens, add the salt, pepper, and oregano (fresh or dried). After the pasta finishes cooking, drain it and top with the sauce before sprinkling it with the pine nuts and feta cheese.

Jerk Chicken and Pineapple Slaw

One more recipe to consider is a full serving of *jerk chicken and pineapple slaw* if you're craving a dinner that's both sweet and tangy. This dinner is great for lowering high blood pressure, along with being free of dairy, sodium, eggs, and nuts. Have a look at all of the ingredients you'll need to put this easy dish together under just half an hour:

- ½ of a pineapple (peeled, chopped, and cored for use)

- 3 heads of thinly sliced baby bok choy

- 2 cups of shredded red cabbage

- 2 teaspoons of jerk seasoning

- 4 teaspoons of packed brown sugar

- 2 teaspoons of all-purpose flour

- 2 tablespoons of apple cider vinegar

- 4 boneless and skinless chicken breast halves (1 to 1 ¼ pounds)

The first step to this dish is prepping the pineapple slaw. For starters, you'll need to mix the pineapple, cabbage, and bok choy in a big bowl. In a smaller bowl, mix together the 2 teaspoons of brown sugar and the cider vinegar; drizzle this new mixture over the bok choy concoction before setting the finished result to the side.

The second step is to take out a large resealable plastic bag and combine the jerk seasoning, flour, and the last 2 teaspoons of brown sugar. Then add in the chicken breast halves and shake them around in the bag to coat. Afterwards, grease up a 12-inch skillet or grill pan and add the coated chicken.

Let the chicken cook for 8 to 12 minutes over medium-high heat, preferably at 170 degrees Fahrenheit, until it's no longer a pink color. Turn the chicken around once it's halfway finished cooking. Once it's complete, put the chicken atop a cutting board and slice it up to eat along with the pineapple slaw.

This chapter has gone over several different meal recipes in length, highlighting some of the nutrient-rich ingredients that help decrease your blood pressure. Not only do they provide several different supplements to bolster your health, but many of them are also easy and quick to make, taking only a little bit of time out of your schedule.

Along with all these nutritious recipes, there are also different kinds of plans or schedules you can follow to motivate you towards eating healthier foods that decrease your blood pressure. Read on to the next chapter to get some good ideas on the various types of diet plans you can implement into your everyday routine.

Chapter 2:

Planning Your Diet

In the previous chapter, we shared various recipes that are beneficial for lowering your blood pressure. These ideas help start you off with a diet that's both simple and quick to implement. However, there are also many different kinds of dietary plans that don't require much cooking, focusing mainly on food types that decrease blood pressure and improve your health. In this chapter, we'll go over some easy and fast diet strategies to help you better manage your blood pressure.

The DASH Diet

One example of a dietary strategy to decrease your high blood pressure is known as the Dietary Approaches to Stop Hypertension, or the DASH diet for short. In an article on WebMD, MD James Beckerman explains how the DASH diet consists of four main categories. The first category involves eating more fruits and vegetables in your daily diet, as well as cutting back on low-fat dairy products. The second category includes steering clear of any foods that contain high amounts of cholesterol, trans fat, and saturated fat. The third category emphasizes eating more foods high in whole grains, along with eating more nuts, poultry products, and fish. The fourth and final category of the DASH diet suggests limiting how much sugar, sodium, and red meat you take in. Beckerman explains how those who participated in the DASH diet were successful in lowering their high blood pressure in the span of just two weeks. There's another variation of this diet, known as the DASH Sodium diet, which involves reducing how much sodium you consume to ⅔ teaspoon each day. Individuals who participated in this dietary method also managed to lower their blood pressure.

When you decide to try out the DASH diet, the first thing to keep in mind is you're only permitted a specific amount of servings per day from different groups of food. How many servings you need is different for every person, because everyone has a different number of categories they need for their daily routines. Beckerman's article explains how you can change up your daily diet when you start the primary DASH diet, such as only taking in 1 teaspoon of sodium daily. After your body begins to adjust to your new diet, decrease your sodium intake even more to only ⅔ teaspoon each day. The sodium you eat in various food products or homemade meals also counts toward these decreased sodium amounts.

If you're struggling to think of ways to add fruits to your diet, the DASH diet provides some useful tips.You can use dried or canned fruits, ideally free of any added sugars. For vegetables, consider having them as a side dish for all your lunches or dinners. Include dry beans or more vegetables as a central part of your daily diet. You can also replace whatever cream or full-fat products you'd normally drink and stick to drinking skim or low-fat dairy products.

When it comes to limiting the amount of meat you consume, the DASH diet recommends 6 pounds of red meat per day at most. Another suggestion is to only use half the amount of butter, salad dressing, or margarine you would normally use and switch them out with low-fat or fat-free condiments. Furthermore, rather than snack consistently on chips and sweetened products, focus on unsalted nuts or pretzels. Other good substitutes include unsalted and butter-free popcorn, low-fat and fat-free yogurt, frozen yogurt, raisins, and raw vegetables. Carefully examine food labels while selecting products with low amounts of sodium.

The following is a list of how many servings from each food category the DASH diet suggests that you have each day:

- For grains, stick to 7 to 8 servings daily

- For fruits, it should be 4 to 5 servings daily

- For vegetables, the total amount ought to be 4 to 5 servings daily

- For fat-free or low-fat dairy products, it should be 2 to 3 servings daily

- For meat, poultry, and fish, you should have 2 or less servings per day

- For oils and fats, stick to 2 to 3 servings daily

- For sweets, limit yourself to only having less than 5 servings total every week

If you happen to be confused on how much a 'serving' is, Beckerman elaborates how much of a specific food group is considered a serving.

- ½ a cup of cooked pasta or rice

- A single slice of bread

- ½ a cup of cooked fruits and vegetables or 1 cup of raw fruits and veggies

- 3 ounces of cooked meat

- 8 ounces of milk

- 3 ounces of tofu

- 1 single teaspoon of olive oil or other oils (Beckerman, 2021)

Sodium Intake

In another article of his, Beckerman explains how reducing your daily salt intake is another great strategy for lowering high blood pressure. He explains the American Heart Association suggests people should only have less than 2,500 milligrams of sodium every day. If they happen to have naturally high blood pressure, or if they already have diabetes or kidney disease, the maximum amount of sodium they should consume is 1,500 milligrams per day or less. That counts towards anything they eat, ranging from small snacks to big dinners. There are a handful of useful tips people can try out to lower their salt intake and blood pressure.

- Train yourself to resist the temptations of grabbing your salt shaker. This is done to avoid putting salt, or more of it, on meals sitting at the table—the American Heart Association states table salt contains 40% sodium (Beckerman, 2021).

- Consider cutting back on how many packaged and processed foods you eat, because these products contribute the most amount of sodium to people's diets.

- Closely scan the labels of packaged foods. When it comes to crackers, cereals, canned veggies, pasta sauces, or any other foods, look for options that are low in salt or sodium.

- When you go out to restaurants, ask your waiter about salt that's added to meals and request for the chefs to lower or remove salt from your dish.

Check if your local eateries post the nutritional information of their dishes so you can see how much sodium is included with each serving. It's also recommended to keep an eye out for any low-sodium options. Also, if you happen to be cooking on your own, you should only add salt at the very end if you need it for whatever recipe you're making (Bekcerman, 2021).

An article written by Cleveland Clinic goes into detail about the different types of food one should avoid or favor when it comes to high blood pressure. For example, foods that are low in fats and calories are safe to consume. The article also recommends you should guse vinegar, herbs, spices, lemon, or other fruit juices to add more flavor to your meals instead of salt. You should avoid using copious amounts of butter, oils, dressings, or margarine with your dishes. Cleveland Clinic also lists many different foods you should incorporate into your diet to lower hypertension. Some options include lean meat, cooked hot cereal, chicken and turkey with no skin, fresh or frozen fruits and veggies, plain pasta and rice, and 'prepared' convenience food low in salt. Other ideal choices include unsalted seeds from squashes, pumpkins, or sunflowers.

The article also explains the key difference between salt and sodium. Salt is a chemical compound made of sodium and chloride, while sodium is a mineral. There are different variations of sodium that exist in different foods, such as monosodium glutamate, or MSG, which is found in most Chinese dishes. Some other foods high in sodium include processed foods like ham and other lunch meats. There are also dried soup mixes or soup cans, boxed potato mix, or foods marinated or pickled in brine. Other ways you can alter your diet to decrease your sodium intake are to broaden your variety of foods, steer clear of consuming alcohol, or eat more foods with high amounts of dietary fiber. These include certain pastas, cereal, or fresh fruit and veggies.

To put things into better perspective, Cleveland Clinic lists several comparisons of how much sodium is found in different food options.

- Dairy

  - Whole milk contains 120 milligrams of sodium per cup

  - 1% or skim milk has 125 milligrams per cup

  - Swiss cheese has 75 milligrams per ounce

  - Cheddar cheese holds 175 milligrams per ounce

- Vegetables

  - Frozen or canned veggies have 55 to 470 milligrams per ½ cup

  - Salt-free canned veggies have less than 70 milligrams per ½ cup

  - Canned tomato juice holds about 660 milligrams for every ¾ cup

- Meat, fish, and poultry
  - Fresh meat contains less than 90 milligrams per 3 ounces
  - Shellfish has 100 to 325 milligrams per 3 ounces
- Cereals, breads, pasta, and rice
  - 1 slice of bread holds 110 to 175 milligrams of sodium
  - Cooked and unsalted cereal contains less than 5 milligrams for every ½ cup
  - Instant cooked cereal has 180 milligrams of sodium per packet
  - Many different canned soups have 600 to 1,300 milligrams per cup
- Convenience foods
  - Frozen and canned main dishes have 500 to 1,570 milligrams of sodium for every 8 ounces and they can also have large amounts of saturated fat (Cleveland Clinic, 2022)

Pritikin Plan

The DASH diet is not the only method you can abide by to decrease your blood pressure. There's another simple meal plan you can use to decrease your blood pressure, developed by the Pritikin Longevity Center. In her article for the Pritikin Program, journalist Eugenia Killoran describes a "5-Day Super-Simple" meal plan that's helpful to fight against both blood pressure and weight loss. She also explains how this diet is very low in sodium, while still being rich with flavor.

Day 1

The breakfast for the first day of the diet should consist of 1 cup of fat and sugar-free vanilla Greek yogurt with half of a cantaloupe. You can get creative and scoop out the cantaloupe's insides and mix it in with the yogurt for extra flavor. This breakfast meal should also include a whole-wheat English muffin with a sugar-free applesauce spread. For a drink, you can choose between coffee, tea, or nonfat or soy milk.

Then comes the mid-morning snack, depending on how hungry you are at the moment. You can choose either two apricots or 1 cup of sugar snap peas, the latter of which you can dip into a side of wasabi. Come lunch time, the plan explains how to make a giant chopped salad with "Pritikin-style" Thousand Island dressing. You can use whatever vegetables you want and put them into a crisper. Some of the best ones to use, recommended by guests at Pritikin, include the following:

- carrots

- broccoli florets

- radishes

- red onions

- cauliflower florets

- tomatoes

- cucumbers

- Romaine lettuce

Next, chop up your veggies with a knife or salad chopper and toss them all into a large bowl. Place the chopped veggies into the fridge to keep them cool while you get started on the dressing. This particular Thousand Island dressing includes the following ingredients:

- ¾ cup of fat-free Greek yogurt

- ¾ cup of low-sugar and low-sodium ketchup

- ½ cup of fat-free sour cream

- ½ teaspoon of garlic powder

- ½ teaspoon of dry oregano

Blend together all of these ingredients until the texture becomes creamy and smooth enough. Once that's done, keep it in the fridge for four days, or less depending on when each of your ingredients expire. Along with your lunch, you should also include a ½ whole-wheat bagel with nonfat ricotta cheese spread and a sliced pluot, which is a hybrid of a plum and an apricot.

If you want a mid-afternoon snack, you should opt for a bowl of cherries. Once it's time for dinner, the Pritikin Plan suggests seared salmon with blueberry balsamic bliss and quinoa, along with a big baby greens salad with basil and strawberries. For the blueberry bliss part of the salmon, boil ¼ cup of balsamic vinegar and 1 cup of fresh or frozen or thawed blueberries in a saucepan over the stove. Reduce the heat as you cook and keep stirring it, until the heat reduces the mixture to half the amount it was before ladling the mixture over the seared salmon. As for the quinoa, all you need is to mix together some quinoa and water in a microwavable bowl, and add some sodium-free seasoning and onion flakes too before heating it up in the microwave for 4 minutes.

If you're in the mood for dessert, the plan recommends a savory watermelon snow cone. The night before dinner, puree 6 cups of chopped seedless watermelons in a blender and pour the contents in an airtight container to put in the freezer. Let the frozen fruit thaw before serving it in a cup or cone (Killoran, 2021).

Day 2

The Pritikin Plan goes on to Day 2. Breakfast for this second day should start off with a bowl of steel-cut oatmeal, preferably from Starbucks. The oatmeal should be made with soy or nonfat milk and free of any packets of brown sugar, raisins, or caloric nuts. Sliced bananas are a healthier substitute. You can also have an apple or orange on the side. For a drink, the plan recommends an unsweetened vanilla latte, made with nonfat or soy milk. If you're up for a mid-morning snack, you should lean towards a salad bar at your local supermarket, such as Whole Foods.

For lunch, the meal plan recommends a veggie sandwich from restaurants like Subway. The bread should be scooped out to greatly reduce your sodium intake. If you're feeling up for a mid-afternoon snack, you should buy a baked potato from Wendy's, since potatoes are low in calories and you can get one with pico de gallo or sour cream. Your dinner should consist of seafood at a steakhouse, steamed vegetables, and other healthy side dishes like a side salad or corn on the cob. Top the day off with a basket of fresh fruit for dessert (Killoran, 2021).

Day 3

For Day 3, the breakfast according to your meal plan should include oatmeal with soy or nonfat milk and fresh berries. You can also choose between having tea or coffee to drink with it. If you're still hungry for a mid-morning snack, you should opt for a bowl of heirloom tomato gazpacho soup. Here's a list of everything you'll need to put together this simple soup:

- 2 diced seedless heirloom tomatoes

- 2 cups of low-sodium veggie juice

- 1 teaspoon of ground coriander

- 1 teaspoon of picked and chopped Italian parsley

- ¼ cup of minced Vidalia onions

- 1 teaspoon of minced garlic

- ½ a minced jalapeno pepper

- ½ cup of peeled and minced and seeded cucumber

- ½ a minced and seeded red bell pepper

- 2 tablespoons of thinly-sliced purple basil (optional)

The process of making this soup is very simple; mix everything except the basil into a large bowl, and refrigerate it for 20 minutes. Pour the finished soup into smaller bowls and sprinkle the basil on top if you wish.

Next, the meal plan states you should make a tomato and peach salad for lunch. Just cut up 2 peaches and 2 large ripe tomatoes into a bowl and drizzle them with aged balsamic vinegar, lemon juice, and a teaspoon of walnut oil. Then toss in ground pepper and some chopped walnuts to top it off. Along with the salad, you can have a side of corn on the cob.

If you feel like having a snack in the mid-afternoon, enjoy a cup of nonfat Greek yogurt with ½ a banana and raspberries. For a drink, you should make a cup of lemonade with iced water and freshly squeezed lemons.

The dinner course for the third day of this plan will be a veggie burger with a whole-wheat bun and grilled vegetables. The veggie patties you'll use only have half the amount of calories that regular red meat patties have and are lower in sodium. It's also important to look for low-sodium options for whole-wheat buns to reduce the risk of high blood pressure. Some good choices of veggies to grill for your veggie burgers include:

- summer squash

- zucchini

- asparagus

- portobello mushrooms

- bell peppers

- red onions

Before you grill, sprinkle the veggies with all-purpose salt-free seasoning and lightly spray them with oil spray. If you want, you can grill enough of the vegetables to save some leftovers for the next day of your meal plan.

After topping your veggie burger with the grilled vegetables of your choosing, you can also use low-sodium Dijon mustard as an ideal condiment.

Once you're done and feel like having dessert, you can use the grill again to cook some pineapple slices. Grill them for 5 minutes over a medium-high flame on both sides. For extra flavor, sprinkle some cinnamon onto the pineapples half an hour before you grill them. You can also put some fat-free sour cream and vanilla extract on top of them (Killoran, 2021).

Day 4

On Day 4 of the Pritikin Plan, you should start the day with a breakfast of scrambled egg whites with grilled veggies and nonfat ricotta cheese. If you have enough, you can use the leftover grilled vegetables from last night's dinner as a side dish. You can even drizzle a little hot sauce on top, especially low-sodium options like Tabasco. Another side dish to have with your eggs is 1 or 2 whole-wheat toast slices. If you're feeling up for it, you can also break your toast into miniature "bowls" and put the egg whites, grilled veggies, and ricotta cheese on them. For a drink, you can pick either tea or coffee.

If you're still hungry around mid-morning, a good snack recommended by the meal plan is a cup of fruit salsa. Some tasty suggestions include berries, melons, and mangos. Chop up the fruit before tossing them into a big bowl, along with chopped cilantro, onions, and squeezed lime.

Later for lunch, you should make a Big Farmer's Market salad. Start by mixing several different fruits, veggies, and produce. Then, you can use either balsamic vinegar or the fruit salsa from earlier as dressing. Along with the salad, you should also try the curry hummus dip. Use the following ingredients to make your dip:

- ¼ cup of chopped onions

- 1 tablespoon of chopped garlic

- 1 diced tomato

- 1 teaspoon of grated ginger

- ½ teaspoon of ground cumin

- ½ teaspoon of ground coriander

- 1 tablespoon of salt-free Caribbean curry powder

- ½ teaspoon of chopped thyme leaves

- 2 cups salt-free garbanzo beans, cooked and drained

- 1 tablespoon of Pritikin all-purpose seasoning

Add the tomatoes, garlic, and onions in a medium-sized nonstick pan and saute them over medium heat for 3 minutes. Throw in the cumin, ginger, thyme, coriander, Caribbean curry powder, and Pritikin seasoning. Cook the mixture on low heat for 8 minutes.

Next, throw in the garbanzo beans and cook and stir them for 5 minutes. Pour the entire mixture into a food processor and puree while it's still hot, before leaving it to cool down.

Once it's finished, you can garnish the hummus dip with sliced apples if you want before eating it. You can also make your own all-purpose seasoning out of the herbs you want, if you don't want to buy the Pritikin brand.

Later on in the mid-afternoon, you can snack on ½ cup of cottage cheese with sliced nectarines. Cottage cheese only has about ⅓ of the sodium that many of us need to have per day. Stick to low-sodium nonfat options when looking for cottage cheese.

For dinner, the meal plan suggests making mahi-mahi ceviche. Luckily, this recipe doesn't require the use of your stove. You first need to cut 1 pound of mahi-mahi into thin and short pieces before tossing them into a large glass bowl. Other ingredients to add to this bowl include:

- ½ cup of lime juice
- ½ cup of chopped and seeded tomatoes
- 1 minced and seeded habanero pepper
- 1 teaspoon of minced garlic
- ground pepper to taste

Toss the concoction in the bowl to coat the mahi-mahi, and top with small sliced red onions. Cover them up in plastic wrap and store them in the fridge for 1 hour. After an hour, take them out and stir them around to mix in the red onions, and put them back in the fridge for 1 more hour.

As a side dish, make yourself some whole-wheat pasta alla checca. Use a large pasta serving bowl to toss around 2 pounds of diced tomatoes, crushed garlic, red pepper flakes, dried oregano, and torn basil leaves.

The only thing you need to cook is the pasta and add it into the serving bowl. Stir the pasta in with the mixture before placing into a smaller bowl. You can even sprinkle the smaller bowl with soy, veggie, or reduced-fat Parmesan cheese.

At the end of Day 4, you can enjoy a dessert of "Perfectly Pritikin" ice cream. The meal plan explains that you can use an appliance called a 'Yonanas' to turn fruit into a frozen dish resembling ice cream. All you need to do is freeze some ripe bananas, thaw them out, and insert them and other fruit like mangos into the Yonanas to convert into Pritikin ice cream. You can also put some fresh berries on them if you want (Killoran, 2021).

Day 5

On Day 5, the final day of the weeklong meal plan, begin your routine with polenta and berry puree. First, pour ½ cup of water into a small saucepan and boil it, then pour ½ of polenta into a small mixing bowl.

Whisk the polenta with a ½ of cold water, and then add in ½ cup of boiling water.

After doing so, lower the heat and let the mixture simmer for 3 to 4 minutes while stirring it occasionally. Then top it with the berries you pureed in a blender and enjoy. Alongside this sweet dish, you can have a cup of nonfat regular or Greek yogurt with sliced fruit and some coffee or tea.

In the mid-morning, depending on how hungry you still are, you can help yourself to a handful of grapes, which are high in fiber and low in calories.

For lunch, the plan suggests you make some ready-made soup. You can simply use a can of veggie and bean soup or microwave a frozen package. It's important to prevent yourself from purchasing any brands that include salt. Once you start to heat up your soup, throw in some other vegetables and herbs you may have on you.

There's also the option of adding some seasonings like garlic or red pepper flakes. You can even have some sugar-free applesauce as a side dish. If you want, you can enjoy some edamame as a mid-afternoon snack.

The dinner course for the fifth day of your meal plan is easy chicken tacos. To make this dish, use the following:

- 1 cup of chopped onions

- 1 cup of chopped red and green bell peppers

- 1 to 2 teaspoons of salt-free Mexican seasoning

- Pre-cooked chicken breast strips

Throw all these ingredients into a nonstick skillet and saute the mixture for about 2 minutes. As it's cooking, throw in a bag of pre-cooked chicken breast strips (preferably low in sodium) and stir them around for 1 minute until they become warm. Finally, dollop them in corn tortillas that you microwaved on a high setting for 1 to 1 ½ minutes, and put some low-sodium salsa on top.

A healthy side dish to eat with these tacos is some fiesta corn salad. To make this side, mix together the following ingredients in a large mixing bowl:

- 1 can of salt-free kidney beans

- 1 bag of frozen white corn kernels to thaw out

- ½ cup of chopped green bell peppers

- ⅔ cup of low-sodium or salt-free salsa

For dessert at the end of the day, feel free to enjoy some dark chocolate pudding. All you need is some sugar-free, fat-free Jell-O. You can also dress your pudding by scooping it into a small dish of fat-free Greek vanilla ice cream. You can optionally top the dessert dish with some raspberries for extra flavor.

Congratulations: you've successfully completed Pritikin's 5-Day, Super-Simple Meal Plan to help lower your blood pressure! (Killoran, 2021)

In this chapter, we covered a few different food products and how much sodium they hold. This is to help you think about how much of certain foods you should have or what to avoid depending on your blood pressure levels. The more you carefully choose which foods to eat in moderation or avoid entirely, the more you're able to reduce your chances of hypertension.

This chapter discussed the DASH Plan and the Pritikin Program's 5-Day Super-Simple Meal Plan. Both of these noteworthy meal plans provide great recipes you can make that greatly reduce your chances of hypertension. If neither of these dietary strategies are appealing to you, there are always several other different plans you can try out. If anything, the next chapter covers a few other diet plans that might be a better fit for you. Read on to learn about a few more meal plans that are helpful for lowering high blood pressure.

Chapter 3:

Other Diet Options

Other than the DASH diet plan, there are other step-by-step dietary plans that can follow on a weekly basis. In his article for *Diet vs Disease*, dietitian Joe Leech writes about the 7-Day Diet Plan designed to help with high blood pressure. This 7-day meal plan is built precisely for people who are busier than others and helps them prepare for their new diet schedule in advance. It also includes several different healthy recipes, all of which are simple to follow and aren't too complicated to prepare. There's also the additional benefit of these recipes being adjustable to your budget, save for a few certain dishes I will cover later on. The dishes incorporated in this diet are very low in salt, reducing your risk of hypertension. Furthermore, these meals are abundant in nutrients, such as magnesium and potassium, that can help with high blood pressure.

Before you go forward with the 7-Day Diet Plan, Leech states there are a few tips to take into consideration. First, you should talk with a personal dietitian or doctor about this dietary routine. When you open up about the prospect of changing your usual diet, it will be good for you to update those specialists on your personal medical history, any medications you're currently taking, and other factors they need to know about. The second tip is to lean heavily towards water as your main drink. While the meal doesn't explicitly say you need water, it's a good idea to constantly have a bottle of water on you to keep yourself hydrated. You can also use certain brands of coffee or tea unless you happen to be sensitive to caffeine.

The third tip is to stay flexible to changes. The 7-Day Diet Plan may not suit all your personal needs; should this be the case, stay open-minded about switching out or omitting certain ingredients or meals. For example, leave breakfast out of the plan if you don't normally eat it. You should also cook up batches of meals to have prepared, so you can simply reheat them if you're in a hurry. The next tip is to avoid eating junk food and other highly processed food products. The recipes included in this meal plan consist of refined and whole foods that greatly improve your health, and many different types of junk food contain high levels of salt. However, some snacks are still a viable option to include in your diet depending on your particular eating routines. Finally, another thing to consider is that these recipes can provide about 2 to 4 servings. As you prepare and eat these hearty dishes, you're bound to have some leftovers on your hands that you can save for the following day.

Day 1 of 7

Now to get started on the 7-Day Diet Plan. For Day 1, your breakfast should include a bowl of oats with milk and a banana on the side. For lunch, your course will be a Simple Summer salad with balsamic vinaigrette, which should only take 20 minutes to prepare. Here's a list of the ingredients you'll need to put this salad together:

- 3 cups of arugula

- 1 corn ear

- ½ cup of halved cherry tomatoes

- ¼ cup of fresh mozzarella cheese

- 2 hard-boiled eggs

- 3 tablespoons of olive oil

- 2 tablespoons of balsamic vinegar

- 1 clove of minced garlic

- salt and pepper

First, you must steam the corn ear for 5 to 7 minutes before cutting off the cooked kernels and moving them aside. The next step is to prepare the salad dressing by mixing together all the ingredients, minus the corn and arugula, into a large jar and shaking it around. Then place 1 ½ cups of arugula and ½ of each of the mixed ingredients into two smaller serving bowls and enjoy.

The course for dinner later in the day will be a dish of apple pecan chicken. You will need the following to cook this dish to your liking:

- 1 pound of boneless and skinless chicken breasts

- ¼ cup of tightly-packed shredded apples

- ½ cup of chopped pecans

- 3 tablespoons of hummus

- 1 strip of diced bacon (optional)

Start by preheating your oven to 400 degrees Fahrenheit. Then put the shredded apples into a paper towel and squeeze them to remove any leftover moisture. Next, mix the apples, bacon, and hummus into a small bowl. Take the chicken breasts and pat them dry with another paper towel or lightly coat them with flour before putting them onto a baking sheet.

Your next task is to coat the chicken by spreading the hummus mixture onto them, then sprinkling the chopped pecans on top of them, pressing them into the hummus spread. Finally, bake the chicken for 20 minutes or until it cooks thoroughly.

Throughout Day 1, you can also enjoy some snacks like some roasted almonds or cashews, as they have high amounts of magnesium and fiber.

Day 2 of 7

During Day 2 of the dietary plan, your breakfast will be a healthy chocolate peanut butter and banana smoothie bowl, which only takes a total of 5 minutes to make. Here is everything you'll need to make this delicious breakfast to start the day:

- ¼ cup of skim milk
- ½ cup of plain 0% Greek yogurt
- 1 frozen diced banana
- 1 tablespoon of natural peanut butter
- 1 tablespoon of cocoa powder
- ¼ cup of rolled oats
- 1 tablespoon of honey
- ¼ tablespoon of vanilla
- a sliced banana
- cacao nibs
- crushed peanuts

This recipe only consists of two steps. First, mix the peanut butter, cocoa powder, yogurt, frozen banana, milk, honey, vanilla, and oats in a blender or food processor, before pouring the mixture into a bowl. Second, sprinkle the breakfast bowl with the cacao nibs, crushed peanuts, and sliced banana.

Later for lunch, you should eat some canned tuna in water or oil with a side salad. Come dinner time, your meal will be roasted salmon and asparagus.

For any snack options, you are free to have 1 cup of cucumber and carrot sticks, along with some hummus or ricotta cheese.

Day 3 of 7

For Day 3 of the 7-Day Diet Plan, you'll make a grapefruit green smoothie for your breakfast. Not only does this breakfast beverage take a short amount of time to make, but it's also high in vitamins A and C. You'll need these ingredients to make this delicious smoothie:

- ½ cup of plain yogurt (dairy-free also works)
- ¾ cup of almond milk or your choice of non-dairy milk
- ½ a segmented and peeled grapefruit
- 1 cup of frozen or fresh spinach
- ½ teaspoon of ground ginger root or 1 inch of peeled ginger root
- ½ a frozen or fresh banana

The only thing you need to do is peel the grapefruit and slice it into large pieces to put inside the blender, along with all the other ingredients, and puree the mixture until it's smooth enough to drink.

The lunch course for this day will be a quinoa salad with nuts. The first thing you need to do for this salad is to take red and white quinoa and mix them together inside a pot with water. Boil the water before lowering the heat to a simmer for 18 minutes or until the quinoa absorbs it all.

For vegetables, it's highly suggested you use chopped cucumbers, sliced cherry tomatoes, steamed asparagus, chopped zucchini or broccoli (raw or steamed are fine), frozen or fresh corn or peas, chopped bell peppers, sliced radishes, roasted cauliflower, or roasted Brussels sprouts. If none of these choices appeal to you, you can be creative and use any veggies of your choosing.

Whichever vegetables choose, chop them up into bite-sized chunks. The same goes for the greens you choose for the salad, such as spring mix, baby spinach, kale, watercress, pea shoots, or arugula. The next step is to add fresh herbs to the salad. Some great options include parsley, basil, mint, cilantro, dill, or tarragon.

Once that's done, the next ingredient to add to the salad is a choice of fruit. You are allowed to use whatever you prefer, such as dried cranberries or golden raisins. Lastly, be sure to include some type of nuts, whether they be pecans, walnuts, or hazelnuts. For the dressing of this salad, it will need to be:

- Olive oil

- Vinegar

- juice from half a lemon

- 1 tablespoon of Dijon mustard

- salt and pepper

- 1 tablespoon of honey or a few drops of liquid stevia

Some additional ingredients you can also throw into your salad include chickpeas, black beans, or lentils. Once the quinoa is finished boiling, let it cool off as you chop up your veggies and greens.

Then place 1 or 2 cups of the finished quinoa into a large bowl. Toss all the ingredients into the bowl as well. However, put the dressing ingredients into a small Mason jar and shake them together before pouring it over your salad. Finally, you can sprinkle your nuts of choice on top.

Afterwards, it will be time to prepare your dinner in the evening: healthy Chipotle chicken sweet potato skins. This particular recipe takes about 1 hour and 30 minutes to complete, but the results are well worth it. Here are all the things required to cook this dish:

- 3 medium-sized sweet potatoes

- 1 pound of boneless and skinless chicken breasts

- 14 ounces of drained chickpeas (optional)

- 4 tablespoons of olive oil

- 4 cloves of grated or minced garlic

- 2 to 3 chipotle chiles in chopped adobo

- zest of 1 lime

- black pepper

- kosher salt

- 2 teaspoons of chili powder

- 1 teaspoon of onion powder

- 1 teaspoon of dried oregano

- 1 teaspoon of cumin

- 2 cups of chopped baby spinach

- 1 cup of shredded white cheddar

- ¼ cup of chopped cilantro

Preheat your oven to 425 degrees Fahrenheit before pricking your sweet potatoes with a fork. Bake the potatoes directly on the oven rack for 50 to 60 minutes or until they tenderize. Take them out of the oven to cool off as you cook the chicken.

Place the chicken breasts and chickpeas on a baking dish, then gently add in the garlic, chili powder, onion powder, cumin, olive oil, chipotle chiles, oregano, lime zest, and a pinch of salt and pepper to coat the chicken. Place them into the oven to bake for 20 to 25 minutes to completely cook through.

Once the last 5 minutes of cooking arrive, take the chicken out of the oven to sprinkle the spinach and put it back in for 5 minutes to let the spinach wilt. After it's finished baking, shred the chicken with two forks and toss them with the spinach, chickpeas, and any residual oils on the baking sheet.

Scrape the sweet potato skin out of the peel, so you're left with a ½ inch-thick layer of sweet potatoes. Then brush the potato skins with the olive oil and bake them for 5 minutes.

Once they're done, take them out of the oven, stuff them with the chicken, and sprinkle the shredded white cheddar on top. Put the decorated skins back inside the oven to bake for 10 more minutes, and then you can have them with a side of Greek yogurt and cilantro.

For your snack options during this day, the meal plan suggests having 5 to 7 ounces of plain Greek yogurt with a small banana.

Day 4 of 7

For Day 4 of this plan, start off your morning with a breakfast of apple walnut quinoa. Later on, during lunch, the plan states that you stick to pumpkin soup. The list of ingredients you'll need for this particular recipe is short yet straightforward:

- 1 pumpkin weighing about 17.6 ounces

- 2 whole onions with their skin

- 1 whole knob of garlic

- salt and pepper

- 6 ¼ cups chicken or vegetable stock

First, cut up the pumpkin into small wedges and then cut off the skin. Then cut the wedges into smaller pieces, since their short size will make them cook quicker. Place the pumpkin wedges on a nonstick baking sheet and let them warm up for 30 to 40 minutes, with your oven at 350 degrees Fahrenheit.

Take them out of the oven once their texture has softened. Next up, place a large saucepan on the stove to get the soup ready. To do this, take the onions out of their skins and toss them into the pan. Do the same for the garlic knob. After disposing of the skins, put the pumpkin wedges inside the saucepan. Once you've done so, put 6 ¼ cups of chicken or vegetable stock inside the pan and begin to boil the mixture for 5 minutes.

Finally, take the saucepan off the stove and stir the mixture together with a stick blender to smooth it out. For extra flavor, add 1 tablespoon of curry paste or sprinkle dry herbs on the soup. You can even drizzle the pumpkin mixture with maple syrup before baking it to caramelize the vegetables.

Later in the day, help yourself to a serving of green lentil and walnut bolognese with pasta for your dinner course.

If you're craving snacks at any point throughout this day, you should have some roasted almonds or cashews.

Day 5 of 7

Once Day 5 of the meal plan arrives, your breakfast should consist of a chocolate peanut butter smoothie. This is a good food choice to start the day as it's high in protein and staves off cravings for snacks later in the day. You only require a few ingredients to make this sweet and healthy drink:

- 1 banana to cut into chunks and freeze

- 3 tablespoons of cocoa

- 2 tablespoons of peanut butter

- 1 tablespoon of honey (optional)

- ¾ cup of plain Greek yogurt

- ¾ cup of milk

All you have to do is throw everything into a blender, switch it on at a low setting while slowly raising it to a higher speed, and blend it together until it's smooth enough to drink.

Later for lunch, your dish will be a roasted sweet potato salad. Here are all the ingredients you need to get started:

- 1 medium-sized sweet potato, cut into 1-inch sized pieces
- 1 half of a red or yellow bell pepper to seed and dice
- 1 half of a minced jalapeno
- 1 clove of minced garlic
- a few tablespoons of chopped red onions
- zest of 1 lemon or lime
- 1 cup of black beans
- ⅓ cup of chopped fresh cilantro

Start by preheating your oven to 400 degrees Fahrenheit before placing the sweet potatoes, bell peppers, garlic, and jalapenos onto a baking sheet. Drizzle everything with olive oil, toss them to coat, spread the ingredients into an even layer, and sprinkle salt and pepper on them.

Roast and turn them a few times for 30 to 40 minutes or until the potatoes' corners turn brown. Take the potato mixture out of the oven and keep it on the pan until it's time to mix the other ingredients. Then, mix in the red onions, black beans, lemon or lime zest, and cilantro into a small bowl.

Add in the sweet potato mixture and drizzle some more olive oil. Finally, season it with salt, pepper, and honey, and you're done!

If you want a snack at all, the plan recommends that a banana should suffice.

Day 6 of 7

For Day 6, you can have any breakfast of your choosing! But for lunch, according to the meal plan, you should make fresh spring rice-paper rolls. You can customize these rolls with whatever vegetables or other healthy ingredients you desire, including the rice wrappers and the dipping sauce. To help you get started, some veggies you can use include carrots, red cabbage, avocado, romaine lettuce, and cilantro.

Vegetables such as these contain high levels of nutrients and antioxidants that improve various areas of your health, especially blood pressure. You should then chop up your ingredients and lay out a small assembly line with your rice wrappers.

Once it's time to make dinner, your main course will be grilled spicy honey lime chicken kebabs. The ingredients you'll need include the following:

- 1 pound of skinless boneless chicken breasts (cubed and trimmed)

- ¼ cup of honey
- 1 teaspoon of Chipotle powder
- 2 teaspoons of garlic powder
- juice from 1 lime
- whatever veggies you want (peppers, tomatoes, zucchini, etc.)

Your first step is to soak the skewers in water to stop them from burning. Next, customize the order you place the chicken and veggies on the skewers before marinating them all in lime juice, garlic powder, honey, and Chipotle powder for a couple of hours. Once that's done, grill the kebabs over a charcoal grill until they're thoroughly cooked.

If you're in the mood for snacks, the plan suggests you try some healthy microwave popcorn.

Day 7 of 7

You have now entered the final day of the dietary plan. For breakfast, you'll be making creamy coconut milk quinoa pudding. These are the only things you'll need to make this small yet savory dish:

- ¾ cup of uncooked quinoa to rinse and drain
- 14 ounces of light coconut milk

- 2 tablespoons of 100% pure maple syrup

- 1 teaspoon of vanilla extract or vanilla bean paste

- 1 tablespoon of whipped cream and blueberries

If you don't have maple syrup, you can swap it with honey. Begin pouring the coconut milk and quinoa into a small saucepan and boil it over high heat. Then lower the heat to medium-low and add in maple syrup or honey and vanilla.

Keep cooking and stirring the mixture for 30 minutes to make it light and creamy enough to be considered pudding. Pour the mixture into another bowl and put it in the fridge for a few hours. Once it's finished, place a ½ or ¾ cup inside a smaller dish and dig in.

You can also use whipped cream, blueberries, or even nuts to garnish the pudding. Once it's time to make lunch, you can pick whatever you want, whether it's leftovers or going out to grab a bite.

For your last dinner of this meal plan, you'll make a bibimbap nourishing bowl. Bibimbap means "mixed rice" in Korean and has plenty of vegetables high in protein. This is the extensive list of ingredients you need:

- ½ cup of brown rice

- 1 cup of water

- 3 tablespoons of olive oil

- a pinch of salt

- 6 ounces of plain tofu

- 2 cups of chopped spinach or swiss chard with no stems

- 2.65 ounces of peeled rainbow carrots

- 2.29 ounces of julienned courgette

- 2 eggs

- 0.14 ounces of green onions

- 1 tablespoon of sesame seeds (optional)

Put the brown rice and a pinch of salt in a saucepan and boil it with water. Cook the rice at a low heat until it completely absorbs all the water.

Meanwhile, drain and wrap the tofu in a paper towel, before putting a plate or other heavy object on top of the tofu and let it drain for 15 more minutes. Once the tofu is pressed enough, cut it into medium rectangle shapes and coat salt on both its sides. Then put them in a hot grill pan and grill them for 5 minutes on each side until they become golden brown and crispy.

Heat up 2 tablespoons of olive oil in a skillet and saute the swiss chard or spinach, zucchini, and carrots one at a time with salt until they tenderize. The chard or spinach should take 5 to 7 minutes, the carrots should take 5 minutes, while the zucchini ought to take 2 to 4 minutes. If you want to include eggs, fry them with a tablespoon of olive oil and add another pinch of salt.

Once that's finished, put the cooked rice into two bowls and garnish them with the tofu and veggies before finishing the ensemble with the sunny-side up eggs. Finally, garnish the green onions and sesame seeds and stir up the contents in the bowls.

On this last day, if you're craving any snacks, one good choice the plan suggests is sweet potato chips. The plan also suggests you soak the chips in water for 1 hour to remove any starch they have. That way, once you bake them in the oven, they will turn out extra crispy for your enjoyment (Leech, 2019). Once you've finished your dinner at this stage, you will have finished the 7-Day Diet Plan for high blood pressure.

Other Snack Choices

There are a few other great snack options the plan recommends as well, if you don't happen to prefer any of the aforementioned ones in the other seven days. One tasty choice to make is a simple strawberry and banana smoothie. You only need four ingredients to prepare this healthy drink for yourself:

- 6 ounces of vanilla yogurt
- 1 ripe banana
- ½ cup of sugar-free coconut milk
- ½ cup of frozen strawberries

Place all the ingredients into a blender and mix them together until it becomes smooth enough to drink. If you want to, you can even switch out the strawberries for a different fruit to produce a different smoothie.

Another good choice for a snack is a serving of banana bread. This snack also needs just four ingredients and only takes a short amount of time to bake:

- 3 bananas

- 3 eggs

- 1 ½ teaspoon of baking powder

- 1 cup of plain or wholemeal plain flour

First, preheat your oven to 356 degrees Fahrenheit. Meanwhile, blend the bananas until they become smooth in texture. Then, whisk the eggs in a bowl before adding baking powder, blended bananas, and flour. Avoid excessively whisking the batter mixture, otherwise it will become rubbery. Once you're done, pour the batter into a pan lined with baking paper and place it in the oven to bake for 30 minutes.

Optionally, you can add ½ cup of cocoa to the batter to give your banana bread a chocolate taste. Or, you can toss in 1 teaspoon of cinnamon. You can even top your banana bread batter with sliced apples before popping it in the oven.

Either way, you can get creative with these snack ideas by exchanging ingredients, just like the recipes in the main 7-Day Diet Plan. This can make lowering your blood pressure a fun process as the days go by.

In this chapter, we've discussed the 7-Day Diet Plan in extensive detail. For each of the seven days of this plan, you would have to adhere to certain kinds of dishes and meals, while staying away from other dishes that are high in sodium. By sticking to this seven day plan, you'll be able to enjoy several different meals that pack a large amount of nutrients and proteins, improving your health and decreasing your blood pressure.

Conclusion

Hopefully, by this point, you've managed to find at least one healthy recipe that sticks out the most to you. Throughout each of the individual chapters, we covered dozens of different healthy recipes that are fast to make and have tons of nutritional value. We discussed recipes such as veggie and hummus sandwiches, Chinese ginger beef stir-fry with baby bok choy, beef and bean sloppy joes, seared scallops with white bean ragu and charred lemon, and so many more. Each of these delicious recipes are not only packed with flavor, but also have individual ingredients consisting of fruits or vegetables essential for decreasing your blood pressure.

We also summarized the different types of meal plans and dietary routines you can exercise to cut back your chances of hypertension. One such strategy involves the Dietary Approaches to Stop Hypertension (DASH), which is comprised of four categories:

- Eat more fruits and vegetables and reduce the number of low-fat dairy products you eat.

- Stay away from foods that have high amounts of cholesterol, trans fat, or saturated fat.

- Eat more fish, nuts, poultry products, and foods with whole grains.

- Cut back on how much sodium, red meat, sugary foods, and drinks you have on a daily basis.

The Pritikin Longevity Center's 5-Day Super-Simple Meal Plan is another option. This method covers an entire work week of sticking to a certain eating schedule. Thankfully, many of these dishes are high in protein and nutrients you'll need to decrease hypertension. Some of these recipes include polenta with berry puree, mahi-mahi ceviche, and even Subway veggie sandwiches. Not only do you have access to a wide variety of dishes, but they are also quick and simple to have, so you don't have to worry so much about cooking time.

Finally, there is the 7-Day Diet Plan by Joe Leech. Some of the standout recipes included in this meal plan are the chocolate peanut butter and banana smoothie bowls, simple summer salad with balsamic vinaigrette, fresh spring rice-paper rolls, and coconut milk quinoa pudding. Each of these recipes vary in terms of how exotic they are and the types of healthy ingredients they're made with to combat high blood pressure.

If you've read through the entirety of this book and are either suffering from hypertension—or want to figure out how to maintain a regular level of blood pressure—utilize everything we've covered thus far. There's a huge variety of recipes at your disposal that you can cook, along with some useful diet strategies to keep you on a healthy diet to maintain a normal blood pressure. By following these dietary methods and sticking to eating healthier dishes, you'll be able to improve your blood pressure and lower the chances of developing hypertension or other health conditions that are dangerous for your health. Start applying the methods and recipes discussed in this book today to lower your blood pressure and live a healthier and happier lifestyle.

References

Ball, M. J. S. (2020 January 30). 25 Healthy High-Blood Pressure Dinners You Can Make in 25 Minutes. *EatingWell*. https://www.eatingwell.com/gallery/7595054/ healthy-high-blood-pressure-dinners-25- minutes/

Beckerman, J. (2021 August 6). *Causes of High Blood Pressure*. WebMD. Retrieved March 18, 2022, from https://www.webmd.com/hypertension- high-blood-pressure/guide/blood-pressure- causes

Beckerman, J. (2021 March 8). *DASH Diet and High Blood Pressure*. WebMD. Retrieved March 15, 2022, from https://www.webmd.com/hypertension-high- blood-pressure/guide/dash-diet

High Blood Pressure Diet: Foods to Eat & to Avoid. (n.d.). Cleveland Clinic. Retrieved March 15, 2022, from https://my.clevelandclinic.org/health/articles/ 4249-hypertension-and-nutrition

Killoran, E. (2021 February 22). *Super-Simple Meal Plan For Blood Pressure and Weight Loss*. Pritikin Weight

Loss Resort. Retrieved March 15, 2022, from
https://www.pritikin.com/simple-meal-plan-
blood-pressure

Leech, J. D. (2019 May 24). *7-Day Diet Plan For High
Blood Pressure (Dietitian-Made)*. Diet vs Disease.
Retrieved March 17, 2022, from
https://www.dietvsdisease.org/diet-plan-high-
blood-pressure/#Day_2

McDermott, A. (2019 March 8). *Diastole vs. Systole: A
Guide to Blood Pressure*. Healthline. Retrieved
March 26, 2022, from
https://www.healthline.com/health/diastole-
vs-systole#TOC_TITLE_HDR_1

Physicians Committee for Responsible Medicine.
(2022). *High Blood Pressure*. Retrieved March 18,
2022, from https://www.pcrm.org/health-
topics/high-blood-pressure

Printed in Great Britain
by Amazon